This book was compiled by Daniel Melehi
with the A.I assistance of Inventabot

<u>Dedication</u>

I hope this helps all of my wonderful
readers achieve all their goals in their
business. And I would like to thank my
wonderful wife for all of her continued
support in all my ventures.

May 7 2023

Contents

Chapter 1: Understanding Fibromyalgia

Fibromyalgia is a chronic pain disorder that affects millions of people worldwide. In this chapter, we will explore the definition, symptoms, prevalence, causes, diagnosis, and treatment of fibromyalgia.

SUBCHAPTER 1.1: DEFINITION AND SYMPTOMS

Fibromyalgia is a disorder characterized by widespread musculoskeletal pain, fatigue, and tenderness in localized areas. Other common symptoms of fibromyalgia include headaches, sleep disturbances, stiffness, depression, and anxiety.

Symptoms of fibromyalgia include:

- Chronic, widespread pain that lasts for at least three months
- Tender points in localized areas of the body
- Fatigue and tiredness
- Sleep disturbances
- Cognitive difficulties, including trouble concentrating, forgetfulness, and decreased alertness
- Mood disturbances, including depression and anxiety
- Headaches
- Stiffness

SUBCHAPTER 1.2: PREVALENCE AND CAUSES

Fibromyalgia affects an estimated 2-8% of the global population, and it is most commonly diagnosed in women. The exact causes of fibromyalgia are unknown, but researchers believe it may be linked to genetics, infections, physical or emotional trauma, or a combination of these factors.

Factors that may contribute to the development of fibromyalgia include:

- Genetics
- Infections, such as viral or bacterial infections
- Physical or emotional trauma, including car accidents, surgeries, or abuse
- Abnormal levels of certain chemicals in the brain and nervous system

SUBCHAPTER 1.3: DIAGNOSIS AND TREATMENT

There is no specific test for fibromyalgia, and it can often be challenging to diagnose. Doctors typically diagnose fibromyalgia by ruling out other conditions and assessing the presence of widespread pain and tenderness in localized areas.

Treatment options for fibromyalgia include:

- Medications, including pain relievers, antidepressants, and anti-seizure medications
- Cognitive-behavioral therapy (CBT), a type of talk therapy that aims to help patients change negative thought patterns and behaviors
- Exercise and physical therapy
- Stress reduction techniques, such as meditation or deep breathing
- Acupuncture and other complementary treatments

If you think you may have fibromyalgia, it is essential to see a healthcare professional for an accurate diagnosis and appropriate treatment. Early intervention can help manage symptoms and improve quality of life.

CHAPTER 1: UNDERSTANDING FIBROMYALGIA

Subchapter 1.1: Definition and Symptoms

Fibromyalgia is a chronic disorder that causes widespread musculoskeletal pain, fatigue, and tenderness in localized areas. The pain and tenderness are often accompanied by other symptoms like insomnia, headaches, and mood disturbances. The exact cause of fibromyalgia is still unknown, but researchers believe that it may be related to a combination of genetic and environmental factors. Additionally, certain triggers like infections, physical or emotional trauma, or surgery may exacerbate the symptoms or even trigger the onset of fibromyalgia in some people. Symptoms of fibromyalgia can vary from person to person, but hallmark symptoms include: - Widespread pain: The pain associated with fibromyalgia is typically described as a constant, dull ache that occurs in multiple areas of the body. The pain may be felt in the muscles, joints, or even in the skin. - Fatigue: People with fibromyalgia often report feeling tired or exhausted, even after getting sufficient rest. The fatigue may be so intense that it interferes with daily activities. - Cognitive difficulties: Many people with fibromyalgia report having difficulty with memory, concentration, and other cognitive processes. This brain fog can be frustrating and impact daily life. - Sleep disturbances: Difficulty falling or staying asleep, or waking up feeling unrefreshed is common in people with fibromyalgia. - Tender points: These are localized areas of tenderness around the neck, shoulders, back, and hips. Pressing on these tender points may cause pain. If you are experiencing these symptoms, it's important to speak with your doctor. There are medical conditions that can mimic fibromyalgia, and ruling out those conditions is important to receiving a proper diagnosis. In the next section, we'll discuss how fibromyalgia is diagnosed and treated.

PREVALENCE AND CAUSES

Fibromyalgia affects approximately 10 million people in the United States alone and is more common among women than men. While the exact cause of fibromyalgia remains unknown, research suggests that it may be linked to a combination of physical, psychological, and environmental factors. One theory is that individuals with fibromyalgia have a heightened sensitivity to pain due to a problem in the way their central nervous system processes pain signals. Additionally, genetics may play a role as fibromyalgia seems to run in families and some genes may make individuals more susceptible to developing the condition. Other research has found that traumatic events, such as car accidents or physical or emotional abuse, may increase the risk of developing fibromyalgia. Additionally, infections or illnesses that trigger an immune response may contribute to the development of fibromyalgia. It's worth mentioning that while there is no known cure for fibromyalgia, there are ways to manage the symptoms and improve overall quality of life for those living with this condition. In the next subchapter, we will explore the diagnosis and treatment options available for fibromyalgia sufferers.

DIAGNOSIS AND TREATMENT

Receiving a diagnosis of fibromyalgia can be a huge relief for those who have been struggling with unexplained pain and other symptoms. However, because there is no definitive test for fibromyalgia, diagnosing the condition can be a difficult and lengthy process. The diagnostic process typically begins with a physical exam and a review of the patient's medical history. The doctor may also order blood tests or imaging scans in order to rule out other conditions that can cause similar symptoms. In order to be diagnosed with fibromyalgia, a patient must have experienced widespread pain for at least three months, with no identifiable underlying cause. Additionally, the patient must have experienced pain in at least 11 out of 18 specific tender points on the body. Once a diagnosis has been confirmed, treatment for fibromyalgia typically involves a combination of medication, lifestyle changes, and other therapies. Some commonly prescribed medications for fibromyalgia include antidepressants, which can help alleviate pain and improve sleep, and pain medications, which can help reduce discomfort. Muscle relaxants, anticonvulsants, and other drugs may also be used to address specific symptoms. In addition to medication, patients may also be advised to make lifestyle changes such as improving sleep habits, reducing stress, and engaging in low-impact exercise. Physical therapy, behavioral therapy, and counseling may also be recommended to help patients manage their symptoms and cope with the emotional challenges of living with fibromyalgia. While there is no cure for fibromyalgia, with proper diagnosis and treatment, many patients are able to manage their symptoms and enjoy a good quality of life.

Chapter 2: Navigating Life with Fibromyalgia

Living with fibromyalgia can be a daily struggle. Symptoms can vary in their intensity and can be unpredictable. Coping with daily challenges can seem overwhelming, but it is crucial to find strategies that work for you.

SUBCHAPTER 2.1: COPING WITH DAILY CHALLENGES

One of the biggest challenges of living with fibromyalgia is dealing with the pain and fatigue on a daily basis. Simple tasks that others take for granted, like doing laundry or grocery shopping, can seem insurmountable. It is important to pace yourself and plan ahead. Breaking up tasks into smaller, more manageable pieces can help. Some other strategies that may help include gentle stretching, meditation, and getting enough rest. Exercise can also be helpful, but it should be approached with care. Low-impact exercise, like walking or swimming, can be beneficial. However, it is important to listen to your body and not push beyond your limits.

SUBCHAPTER 2.2: MANAGING FLARE-UPS

Fibromyalgia flare-ups can be triggered by a variety of factors, including stress, changes in weather, and overexertion. When a flare-up occurs, it can be difficult to know how to manage it. One key strategy is to have a plan in place for managing flare-ups. This may include having a backup for important engagements or scheduling downtime for yourself. Taking steps to reduce stress, such as practicing mindfulness or seeking support from friends and family, can also be helpful. It is also important to be prepared for flare-ups. This might mean having a stock of pain relief medication or investing in tools that can help with daily tasks, like a shower chair or a long-handled reacher.

SUBCHAPTER 2.3: BUILDING A SUPPORT NETWORK

Living with fibromyalgia can be lonely, but it is important to remember that you are not alone. Building a support network can be hugely beneficial. Friends and family can be a great source of support, but it can also be helpful to connect with others who know what you are going through. Online forums or support groups can provide a sense of community and can offer tips and advice from those who have experienced similar struggles. It is also worth considering seeking professional support. A therapist can help you manage the emotional impact of living with chronic pain, and a physical therapist can provide tailored exercises to help manage your symptoms. Remember, managing fibromyalgia requires patience and self-compassion. By finding strategies that work for you and building a strong support network, you can learn to live a fulfilling life with fibromyalgia.

SUBCHAPTER 2.1: COPING WITH DAILY CHALLENGES

Living with fibromyalgia can be challenging, as the symptoms can affect a person's daily life. From pain to fatigue to brain fog, fibromyalgia symptoms can impact a person's ability to work, enjoy hobbies, and even complete everyday tasks. Coping with these challenges requires patience, creativity, and a willingness to adapt. One of the most important things a person with fibromyalgia can do to cope with daily challenges is to prioritize self-care. This means taking the time to rest when needed, eating a healthy diet, and engaging in low-impact exercise. It also means managing stress, as stress can worsen fibromyalgia symptoms. Another important aspect of coping with daily challenges is learning to set realistic expectations. This might mean adjusting expectations for work or social activities, recognizing limitations, and asking for help when needed. A variety of coping techniques can also be helpful for managing fibromyalgia symptoms. These might include techniques such as meditation, deep breathing, or progressive muscle relaxation. Gentle massage or heat therapy might also be soothing for muscle pain. It's important to find what works best for each individual person and to be patient with yourself as you adjust to life with fibromyalgia. Over time, it may become easier to manage daily challenges and find a balance that works for you. Remember, coping with fibromyalgia is a journey, and it's important to be kind to yourself along the way. With the right tools and strategies, it is possible to live a full and satisfying life with fibromyalgia.

MANAGING FLARE-UPS

Managing fibromyalgia is a constant battle, and one of the biggest challenges is dealing with flare-ups. These are periods when your symptoms seem to intensify, sometimes for no apparent reason. Flare-ups can disrupt your daily life and cause a lot of discomfort, but there are strategies you can use to manage them. One important step is to identify triggers that may be causing your flare-ups. This can be anything from a change in weather to stress, lack of sleep, or certain foods. Once you have identified your triggers, you can take steps to avoid or minimize them. Another key strategy is self-care. This entails doing things that promote your overall well-being, such as eating a healthy diet, getting enough sleep, and engaging in physical activity that works for your body. Gentle exercises like stretching, yoga, or walking can help ease pain and stiffness, but it's important not to overdo it. When you do experience a flare-up, it's important to manage your symptoms effectively. There may be times when you need to take medication to alleviate pain, but there are also natural remedies you can try, such as hot or cold compresses, aromatherapy, or massage. It's also important to be gentle with yourself and give your body the time and space it needs to heal. Finally, it's important to have a support system in place. Friends, family, or a support group can provide emotional support and help you through tough times. It's important to communicate with those around you about your needs and limitations so they can assist you when needed. By using a combination of self-care, symptom management, and support, you can effectively manage flare-ups and live a full life with fibromyalgia.

BUILDING A SUPPORT NETWORK

Living with fibromyalgia can be challenging, but having a support network can make all the difference. Building a support network can help you cope with daily challenges, provide emotional support, and offer practical assistance when needed. Here are some tips for building a strong support network:

1. Educate Your Loved Ones about Fibromyalgia

Many people may not understand fibromyalgia and what it entails. It's important to educate your friends and family about the condition and how it affects you. By explaining your symptoms, limitations, and needs, you can help them better understand and support you.

2. Join a Support Group

Joining a support group can be invaluable. You get to meet other people with the same condition, share experiences, learn coping strategies, and receive emotional support. There are both online and in-person support groups. Reach out to your doctor or a fibromyalgia organization for recommendations.

3. Seek Professional Help

Depending on your needs, seeking professional help may also be beneficial. A therapist can provide you with emotional support, help you deal with depression and anxiety, and teach coping skills. A physical therapist can help you manage pain and improve your physical function.

4. Connect with the Fibromyalgia Community

The fibromyalgia community is vast and supportive. Connect with online forums, join social media groups, attend community events, and participate in advocacy efforts. Surrounding yourself with people who understand what you're going through can make a huge difference in your journey.

5. Talk to Your Employer

If you're working, it's important to talk to your employer about your condition. They may be able to provide accommodations like flexible hours, a comfortable workspace, or an ergonomic chair. Some employers may also have employee assistance programs that can provide additional resources. Building a support network takes time and effort, but it's worth it. With a strong support system, you can manage your fibromyalgia and live a full life.

Chapter 3: Mental Health and Fibromyalgia

Living with fibromyalgia is not only physically challenging but mentally as well. Studies have shown that those who suffer from fibromyalgia are at a higher risk for developing depression and anxiety. In this chapter, we will explore different ways to manage your mental state while living with fibromyalgia.

SUBCHAPTER 3.1: DEPRESSION AND ANXIETY

Depression and anxiety are two of the most common mental health conditions that coincide with fibromyalgia. Those who have fibromyalgia are more likely than those who don't to develop one or both of these conditions. Depression can cause a range of symptoms from feelings of sadness and hopelessness to fatigue and difficulty concentrating. When combined with Fibromyalgia, these symptoms can become even more severe. Combatting Depression requires seeking professional help through therapy or support groups. Anxiety can cause symptoms such as restlessness, irritability, and trouble sleeping. Managing anxiety while also managing fibromyalgia can be difficult but not impossible. Mindfulness techniques like yoga, meditation, and deep breathing exercises have been proven to help alleviate anxiety symptoms.

SUBCHAPTER 3.2: COPING WITH STIGMA

Unfortunately, fibromyalgia is an invisible disability. People with fibromyalgia may appear fine on the outside but struggle with pain and fatigue on the inside. This can lead to feelings of isolation and stigma from others who may not understand the severity of the condition. It is essential to communicate your symptoms to those around you and explain the difficulties that come with fibromyalgia. Educating yourself on the condition can also help you to better understand and explain fibromyalgia to others.

SUBCHAPTER 3.3: SEEKING THERAPY

Seeking professional help through therapy is a crucial step in managing your mental health while living with fibromyalgia. A therapist can help you identify negative thoughts and feelings, provide coping strategies, and create a plan for managing depression and anxiety. It's important to find a therapist who is familiar with fibromyalgia and can offer support in a way that works for you. In conclusion, managing your mental health while living with fibromyalgia can be challenging, but there are ways to combat the emotional symptoms that come with this condition. By seeking professional help, educating yourself, and practicing mindfulness techniques, it's possible to live a fulfilling life with fibromyalgia.

CHAPTER 3: MENTAL HEALTH AND FIBROMYALGIA

Subchapter 3.1: Depression and Anxiety

Living with fibromyalgia can be a challenging experience, both physically and mentally. In addition to the physical symptoms, people with fibromyalgia may also experience depression, anxiety, and other mental health conditions. Depression is a common mental health condition that can occur in people with fibromyalgia. It is estimated that around 20-30% of people with fibromyalgia also experience depression. The high prevalence of depression in people with fibromyalgia is thought to be related to the chronic pain and other symptoms associated with the condition. Anxiety is another common mental health condition that can occur in people with fibromyalgia. It is estimated that around 50% of people with fibromyalgia experience anxiety. Anxiety may be related to the uncertainty and unpredictability of fibromyalgia symptoms, as well as the need to navigate a complex healthcare system in order to receive proper treatment. Living with depression or anxiety can make it more difficult to manage the physical symptoms of fibromyalgia. Additionally, the physical symptoms of fibromyalgia can in turn worsen depression and anxiety. This can create a vicious cycle that makes it difficult to manage fibromyalgia symptoms and maintain mental health. Fortunately, there are many strategies that can help manage depression and anxiety in people with fibromyalgia. These may include therapy, medication, lifestyle changes, and self-care techniques. It is important for people with fibromyalgia who are experiencing depression or anxiety to seek professional help in order to develop a treatment plan that is tailored to their individual needs. In conclusion, depression and anxiety are common mental health conditions that can occur in people with fibromyalgia. These conditions can make it more challenging to manage the physical symptoms of fibromyalgia, and vice versa. However, with the right treatment plan and strategies, it is possible to manage these conditions and live a fulfilling life with fibromyalgia.

COPING WITH STIGMA

Living with fibromyalgia is not just about coping with the physical pain and discomfort. It's also about dealing with the stigma that often comes with this invisible disability. Sadly, fibromyalgia is still widely misunderstood, and many people who don't have firsthand experience with it have formed misconceptions about the condition. One of the most common stigmas associated with fibromyalgia is that it's "all in your head." This couldn't be further from the truth. As anyone who lives with fibromyalgia will tell you, the pain and other symptoms are very real and can be debilitating. Unfortunately, some people may not understand that just because they can't see the pain or other symptoms, that doesn't mean they don't exist. Another stigma associated with fibromyalgia is that people who have it are just being lazy or trying to get attention. Again, this is simply not true. In fact, many people with fibromyalgia push themselves to their limits every day, despite the pain and other symptoms they experience. It's important to remember that just because someone has an invisible disability, that doesn't mean they're any less deserving of respect or understanding. So, how can you cope with the stigma associated with fibromyalgia? Here are a few tips: - Educate others: Many people who perpetuate fibromyalgia stigma simply don't know any better. By educating others about the condition and its symptoms, you can help break down some of the misunderstandings surrounding fibromyalgia. - Seek support: Support from friends, family, or a support group can be essential when dealing with stigma. Surround yourself with people who understand and believe in you, and don't let the negative comments of others bring you down. - Focus on self-care: Remember that taking care of yourself and your own well-being is a top priority. Be kind to yourself, and don't push yourself too hard when you're not feeling up to it. - Speak up: If someone is being hurtful or spreading misinformation about fibromyalgia, don't be afraid to speak up. Advocating on behalf of yourself and the fibromyalgia community can help break down stigmas and create a more understanding world. No one should have to deal with the added burden of stigma on top of the physical and emotional challenges of living with fibromyalgia. By educating others, seeking support, focusing on self-care, and speaking up, you can help fight stigma and create a more understanding world for those who are living with invisible disabilities.

Helpful Resources

- National Fibromyalgia and Chronic Pain Association

- The Mighty: Fibromyalgia

- UK Fibromyalgia

And remember, by staying informed and advocating for yourself, you can help create a more understanding world for those living with fibromyalgia.

CHAPTER 3: MENTAL HEALTH AND FIBROMYALGIA

Subchapter 3.3: Seeking Therapy

Living with fibromyalgia can take a toll on your mental health and seeking therapy can be an effective way to manage these symptoms. Therapy provides a safe and confidential space for individuals to talk about their experiences and improve their mental health. One common therapy used for fibromyalgia is cognitive-behavioral therapy (CBT). CBT focuses on changing negative thought patterns and behaviors that contribute to pain and other symptoms. It can also help individuals develop coping mechanisms and improve their problem-solving skills. Acceptance and Commitment Therapy (ACT) is another type of therapy that can be beneficial for individuals with fibromyalgia. ACT focuses on accepting difficult thoughts and feelings, while also committing to actions that are consistent with personal values. This can help individuals better manage chronic pain and other symptoms associated with fibromyalgia. In addition to traditional talk therapy, support groups can be a helpful resource for individuals with fibromyalgia. These groups provide a safe and supportive environment for individuals to share their experiences, receive emotional support, and learn from others. It is essential to find a therapist who is knowledgeable about fibromyalgia and understands the unique challenges individuals with this condition face. Ask your healthcare provider for a referral or do your own research to find a therapist who specializes in chronic pain or fibromyalgia. Overall, seeking therapy can be an excellent way to improve your mental health and learn effective coping strategies for living with fibromyalgia. Remember, it's okay to seek help and prioritize your mental health as a crucial part of your overall wellbeing.

Conclusion

In this chapter, we have explored the mental health challenges that individuals with fibromyalgia face. Seeking therapy can be a useful tool for managing these challenges, as it provides a safe and supportive space to address difficult thoughts and feelings. Additionally, support groups can be a source of emotional support and information. Remember, taking care of your mental health is an essential part of living well with fibromyalgia.

Chapter 4: Fibromyalgia and Relationships

Fibromyalgia not only affects the individual with the condition, but it can also have a significant impact on their relationships. In this chapter, we will explore the different challenges that come with managing relationships while living with fibromyalgia and ways to overcome them.

SUBCHAPTER 4.1:
COMMUNICATING WITH
FAMILY AND FRIENDS

One of the most significant challenges that individuals living with fibromyalgia face is communicating their condition with family and friends. It can be difficult to explain an invisible illness, and loved ones may not understand the extent of the individual's pain and fatigue. Communication is key when it comes to managing relationships with fibromyalgia. It's important to ensure that your loved ones understand your condition and how it affects your daily life. You can start by educating them on the symptoms of fibromyalgia and how it affects you specifically. It's important to be open and honest about your limitations, but also try to emphasize what you can do rather than what you can't. It's also essential to communicate your needs clearly. For example, if you have a friend or family member who wants to plan a day out, let them know what you can and cannot do, and suggest alternatives. Remember, your loved ones want to help you, but they may not know how, so don't hesitate to ask for help when you need it.

SUBCHAPTER 4.2: ROMANTIC RELATIONSHIPS

Living with fibromyalgia can be particularly challenging when it comes to romantic relationships. Chronic pain and fatigue can impact intimacy and often put a strain on the relationship. It's essential to communicate with your partner about your condition and how it affects your relationship. It's important to remember that your partner may also be struggling, and it's important to take their needs into consideration. Try to find alternative ways to maintain intimacy, such as cuddling or gentle massages. It's also important to manage your fatigue levels and plan date nights that work for both you and your partner. Lastly, try to focus on the positives. Fibromyalgia can bring couples closer together as they work together to manage the condition. Remember, you are more than your condition, and it's important to focus on the things you enjoy doing together.

SUBCHAPTER 4.3: PARENTING WITH FIBROMYALGIA

Parenting is a full-time job, and living with fibromyalgia can make it even more challenging. The symptoms of fibromyalgia can impact a parent's ability to care for their children, and it's essential to communicate with your partner and children about your condition. It's important to prioritize self-care, as caring for others can take a toll on a person's health. Parents with fibromyalgia should have a support system in place, such as family members or hired help, to assist with childcare. It's also important to be open and honest with your children about your condition. Explain to them what fibromyalgia is and how it affects you. Encourage them to ask questions and be involved in your care. This not only helps them understand your condition but also helps build empathy and care for others. In conclusion, living with fibromyalgia can be a challenge when it comes to relationships, but with open and honest communication, prioritizing self-care, and being proactive, individuals can manage their relationships effectively.

SUBCHAPTER 4.1: COMMUNICATING WITH FAMILY AND FRIENDS

Living with fibromyalgia can be made easier when you have the support of loved ones. While everyone's experience with fibromyalgia is unique, here are some tips that may help you navigate your relationships with family and friends:

Be Open and Honest

Communication is key to maintaining strong relationships. Talk to your loved ones about how fibromyalgia affects your life. Share any limitations or restrictions you may have due to fibromyalgia and let them know how they can support you.

Ask for Help

Don't hesitate to ask for help when you need it. Whether it's for household chores, running errands, or just needing a listening ear, your loved ones may be more than happy to lend a hand.

Set Boundaries

It's important to set boundaries with your loved ones to avoid overwhelming yourself. Let them know when you need space and time to rest, so you don't push yourself too hard.

Find Ways to Connect

Fibromyalgia can make it difficult to participate in activities that you used to enjoy, but there are still ways to connect with your loved ones. Consider finding new hobbies or activities you can do together or finding creative ways to communicate with each other, like through video calls or social media. Remember, it's okay to prioritize your health, and communicating honestly with your loved ones can help them understand and support you on your fibromyalgia journey.

SUBCHAPTER 4.2: ROMANTIC RELATIONSHIPS

Fibromyalgia not only impacts an individual's daily life but also affects their romantic relationships. Being in a relationship with a person living with fibromyalgia requires understanding, empathy, and patience. One of the biggest challenges individuals with fibromyalgia face in their romantic relationships is the physical and emotional limitations they experience. Many individuals with fibromyalgia experience chronic pain and fatigue, which can make it difficult for them to maintain a healthy sex life. It is essential to remember that individuals with fibromyalgia are not just their illness. Therefore, avoiding sexual intimacy due to their condition can be detrimental to their relationship. Communication with your partner is critical in navigating this aspect of your relationship. Discuss your limitations and boundaries and ways to engage in intimacy that work for both parties. It is crucial to establish a support network within your romantic relationship. Your partner should understand the limitations of your condition and be willing to support you when needed. You should not feel like a burden to your partner when asking for help. Support can be as simple as being there to listen, running errands when you are unable to, or accompanying you to appointments. In many cases, fibromyalgia can cause a disconnect in a relationship due to the imbalance of responsibilities. The more able-bodied partner may be taking on more responsibility than they can handle or feel comfortable with, leading to resentment. Equally, the partner with fibromyalgia may feel like they are a burden, which can lead to feelings of guilt and low self-worth. Open communication and acknowledging each partner's strengths and weaknesses can help balance the relationship. Finally, it is crucial to work on the emotional component of the relationship. Fibromyalgia can cause feelings of isolation and depression, which can be detrimental to any relationship. Couples struggling with fibromyalgia should be open to counseling and therapy to improve their relationship's emotional health. In conclusion, fibromyalgia impacts every aspect of an individual's life, including their romantic relationships. Communication, understanding, empathy, and patience are critical to managing a successful relationship while living with fibromyalgia. Working together, couples can navigate the challenges of fibromyalgia and build a stronger relationship.

The Invisible Disability: Living with Fibromyalgia

CHAPTER 4: FIBROMYALGIA AND RELATIONSHIPS

Subchapter 4.3: Parenting with Fibromyalgia

Parenthood is a challenging experience on its own, and dealing with fibromyalgia can make it even more difficult. The fatigue, pain, and brain fog that come with this condition can make it hard to keep up with the constant demands of caregiving. However, with some adjustments and self-care, it is possible to maintain a fulfilling relationship with your children, despite having fibromyalgia. One of the first things you can do is to communicate with your children about your condition, especially if they are old enough to understand. You do not have to go into great detail, but explain that sometimes you might not be as active or energetic as you would like to be. Encourage them to ask questions and be open about your struggles. Another crucial element of parenting with fibromyalgia is self-care. Taking care of yourself is not a luxury but a necessity to be the best parent you can be. This might mean taking breaks throughout the day to rest or engage in low-impact activities. It is also essential to prioritize sleep, eat healthily, and engage in gentle exercises like stretching or swimming. Delegating tasks to other family members or friends can also help lighten the load. If you are having a flare-up, consider asking for help with household chores or transportation to your children's activities. Building a strong support system can help you overcome the challenges of parenting with fibromyalgia. Finally, it is essential to adjust your expectations and be gentle with yourself. Parenting is not a competition, and it is okay to ask for help, take a break, or say no to certain activities. Remember that you are doing the best you can, and your children love and appreciate you for who you are. In conclusion, parenting with fibromyalgia is not easy, but it is doable with proper communication, self-care, delegating tasks, and being gentle with yourself. It is possible to have a fulfilling relationship with your children despite the challenges of fibromyalgia.

Chapter 5: Working with Fibromyalgia

Living with fibromyalgia can be challenging, especially when it comes to managing work responsibilities while dealing with the symptoms of this condition. In this chapter, we will explore the different ways you can manage your job while living with fibromyalgia.

SUBCHAPTER 5.1: ACCOMMODATIONS IN THE WORKPLACE

A workplace accommodation is any change to the work environment or the way things are usually done that allows an individual with a disability to perform their job duties. If you have a disability like fibromyalgia, you are entitled to reasonable accommodations that will enable you to perform your duties. Some typical accommodations could be adjusted work hours, ergonomic furniture, flexible schedules, and telework arrangements. Be sure to speak with your supervisor or HR department to get accommodations that work.

SUBCHAPTER 5.2: NAVIGATING DISABILITY BENEFITS

If you suffer from fibromyalgia and it interferes with your ability to complete your job responsibilities, you may be eligible for disability benefits. These benefits can help provide you with some financial assistance while you are unable to work. When applying for disability benefits, you must provide all relevant medical information that can support your claim about your condition. It can be a lengthy and challenging process, so be sure to review the guidelines and have a medical professional assist you in the application.

SUBCHAPTER 5.3: FINDING FULFILLMENT OUTSIDE OF WORK

Sometimes, it is essential to take a step back from work and focus on other aspects of your life to manage your fibromyalgia effectively. Consider investing time into hobbies or activities that bring you joy. This could be anything from writing to drawing, yoga, or meditation. Additionally, volunteering your time can provide feelings of fulfillment and satisfaction. Not only can it impact your health positively, but it can also serve as a way to help others. Volunteering has been shown to reduce stress and provide a sense of purpose in life.

CONCLUSION

Chronic pain, fatigue, and cognitive difficulties are just some of the challenges of living with fibromyalgia while working. With the right accommodations in place, navigating disability benefits, and finding fulfillment outside of work, you can lead a full and productive life with fibromyalgia in the workplace. It's essential to prioritize your health above all and seek support from loved ones and medical professionals. Remember, you don't have to do it alone.

ACCOMMODATIONS IN THE WORKPLACE

Living with fibromyalgia can be challenging, particularly when it comes to managing work responsibilities. As a chronic condition, fibromyalgia can make it difficult to keep up with the demands of a traditional work setting. However, with the right accommodations, it may be possible for individuals with fibromyalgia to continue working and thriving in their careers. If you have fibromyalgia, it may be helpful to speak with your employer about possible accommodations. Some examples of workplace accommodations for fibromyalgia may include flexible work hours, the ability to work from home, ergonomic office equipment, and designated rest breaks throughout the day. Additionally, it may be useful to create a work environment that is conducive to managing fibromyalgia symptoms. This may include adjusting the temperature in your workspace, using noise-cancelling headphones to reduce sensory overload, or investing in compression gloves or a standing desk to reduce muscle strain and joint pain. There may also be legal protections available to individuals with fibromyalgia who require workplace accommodations. Under the Americans with Disabilities Act (ADA), employers are required to provide reasonable accommodations to individuals with disabilities, including those with fibromyalgia. If you are experiencing difficulty at work due to fibromyalgia symptoms, it may be worth exploring your options for accommodations. By working together with your employer and carefully managing your symptoms, you can continue to succeed and thrive in your career.

SUBCHAPTER 5.2: NAVIGATING DISABILITY BENEFITS

Living with fibromyalgia can be challenging, and sometimes, it may become impossible to continue working. For people with fibromyalgia, navigating disability benefits can be confusing and stressful, but it's important to understand that you have legal rights and options. An important step in this journey is speaking with your doctor and getting medical documentation to support your claim for disability benefits. This documentation should include a detailed description of your symptoms, the impact of your symptoms on your ability to work, your limitations, and any treatments you are receiving. This information will be key to your claim and will help provide proof to the Social Security Administration (SSA) that you cannot work due to your fibromyalgia. When applying for disability benefits, you should be aware that the process is often lengthy, and it may take months or even years to complete. It's essential to be patient, persistent, and prepared for the possibility that your application may be denied initially. It's not uncommon for the SSA to reject the first application, but with additional medical documentation and consultation with a disability lawyer, approval can be obtained. Seeking legal assistance to navigate disability benefits can be helpful. A disability lawyer can help you navigate the application process and speak on your behalf. A lawyer will also help you understand your legal rights, the appeals process if your claim is denied, and what to expect during the hearing process. In addition to Social Security Disability benefits, you may be eligible for private disability insurance offered through your employer or through another plan. It's essential to understand the terms of your insurance policy and what benefits it offers. If your employer has a human resources department, they can often provide you with information and assistance in filing a claim. Navigating disability benefits can be daunting, but with the right knowledge, preparation, and support, you can obtain the benefits you are entitled to. Don't let the process discourage you from seeking the support you need to manage your fibromyalgia and maintain a fulfilling life. Remember, you are not alone, and there is help available to ensure you have the resources you need to live with fibromyalgia. Keep advocating for yourself and others, and together, we can create a better understanding of this invisible disability.

CHAPTER 5: WORKING WITH FIBROMYALGIA

Subchapter 5.3: Finding Fulfillment Outside of Work

Working with fibromyalgia can be an immense challenge, and many patients need to prioritize their health over their careers. However, it is also important to find ways to enjoy life outside of work and maintain a healthy work-life balance. Here are some tips for finding fulfillment outside of work if you have fibromyalgia:

1. Pursue hobbies that you are passionate about

Engage in activities that interest you and that you can comfortably participate in. Finding a hobby that you are passionate about can provide you with a creative outlet and a sense of accomplishment. You can try activities like painting, knitting, or cooking. These activities can stimulate your brain and keep your body active without overworking yourself.

2. Connect with nature

Spending time with nature can have a positive impact on your mental health. Go for walks in the park, hike or even try bird watching. This will give you a chance to unwind and rejuvenate your body and mind.

3. Stay connected with friends and family

Keeping in touch with friends and family can help you feel supported and provide a social outlet. You can visit family members or schedule phone or video calls with friends who live far away. Meeting new people with similar interests can also bring joy to your life.

4. Explore alternative forms of therapy

Alternative forms of therapy such as acupuncture, massage, or meditation may bring some relief. These holistic approaches can complement conventional medicine to manage symptoms like pain, anxiety, and stress.

5. Travel

You can plan a trip to a nearby area or even take a relaxing weekend getaway. Consider accommodations or transportation options that support your comfort level, like booking rooms on the first floor or bringing comfortable pillows. Remember, it is important to prioritize self-care and seek support as you navigate living with fibromyalgia. By taking time to participate in activities that give you joy, you can maintain a balanced and fulfilling life.

Chapter 6: Advocating for Yourself and Others

Living with fibromyalgia can be challenging, but it can be even more challenging when the people around you do not understand your condition. Advocating for yourself and others is crucial in raising awareness and fighting for disability rights. Below are three subchapters that will help guide you in advocating for yourself and others.

SUBCHAPTER 6.1: RAISING AWARENESS

Raising awareness about fibromyalgia is essential in educating people about the condition and the impact it has on individuals. One effective way to raise awareness is by sharing your story with others. This can be done through social media, support groups, or your personal network. Share your struggles, successes, and ways in which you manage your symptoms. Another way to raise awareness is by getting involved in advocacy groups or organizations. These groups work to educate people about fibromyalgia and advocate for disability rights. By joining these groups, you can take part in events, share information, and bring attention to the challenges that people with fibromyalgia face.

SUBCHAPTER 6.2: FIGHTING FOR DISABILITY RIGHTS

One of the biggest challenges for people with fibromyalgia is navigating the disability system. The disability system is often complicated, and it can be challenging to get the help you need. As an advocate, it is important to fight for disability rights. This can include advocating for changes in policies and regulations to ensure that people with fibromyalgia are treated fairly. You can also advocate for more accommodations in the workplace, schools, and other public areas. These accommodations can include things like flexible schedules, ergonomic workstations, and accessible locations. By advocating for accommodations, you are helping to create a more inclusive environment that can benefit everyone, not just those with fibromyalgia.

SUBCHAPTER 6.3: BUILDING A FIBROMYALGIA COMMUNITY

Building a community of individuals who understand what you are going through is essential in managing fibromyalgia. One way to do this is by joining local support groups or online communities. These communities offer a safe space to share your experiences, ask for advice, and connect with others who are dealing with similar challenges. By building a community, you can also create a collective voice that can be used to advocate for better treatment and support for those with fibromyalgia. Together, you can work to raise awareness, fight for disability rights, and create a more supportive and inclusive world.

Conclusion

Advocating for yourself and others is a powerful way to make a positive impact on the world. By raising awareness, fighting for disability rights, and building a community, you can help create a more inclusive and supportive environment for those with fibromyalgia. Remember, you do not have to take on this challenge alone. Reach out to others for support, and together, you can make a difference.

RAISING AWARENESS

Raising awareness about fibromyalgia is crucial for several reasons. Firstly, it will help people understand the condition better. Since fibromyalgia is an invisible disability, people around us may not be aware of the challenges we face every day. When people become more aware of what fibromyalgia is, they may start to empathize with those who are affected. This empathy can lead to more support for those with fibromyalgia. Secondly, raising awareness can help debunk some of the myths and misconceptions surrounding fibromyalgia. For instance, people may believe that fibromyalgia is not a real condition, or that it's caused by psychological factors. By providing accurate information about fibromyalgia, we can dispel these myths and ensure that people have the right understanding of the condition. Thirdly, raising awareness can lead to more resources and research for fibromyalgia. Increased awareness may lead to more funding for research into the causes and treatments of fibromyalgia. It may also lead to more support groups, education programs and advocacy efforts for people with the condition. There are several ways to raise awareness about fibromyalgia. One way is to share our personal stories about living with fibromyalgia. By sharing our experiences, we can help people understand what it's like to live with the condition. We can also share information about fibromyalgia through social media, blogs, and other online platforms. Participating in awareness campaigns and events is another effective way to raise awareness. Many organizations and groups hold events to increase awareness about fibromyalgia, such as Fibromyalgia Awareness Day, which is observed annually on May 12th. By participating in these events, we can connect with others who are affected by fibromyalgia and spread awareness about the condition. In conclusion, raising awareness about fibromyalgia is critical for increasing understanding, dispelling myths and misconceptions, and securing resources and support. By speaking out and participating in awareness campaigns, we can help others understand what it's like to live with fibromyalgia and work towards better outcomes for everyone affected by this condition.

SUBCHAPTER 6.2: FIGHTING FOR DISABILITY RIGHTS

Living with fibromyalgia is no easy feat, especially when it comes to navigating the complicated world of disability rights. For many with fibromyalgia, their condition is often misunderstood and underestimated. It is vital to understand that fibromyalgia is a disability that impacts a person's daily life. Without the proper accommodations, many people with fibromyalgia struggle to participate fully in society. Fighting for disability rights is essential for those with fibromyalgia, and it involves advocating for accessible accommodations, equal rights, and support services. It's important to remember that fighting for disability rights is not just a one-person job. Many advocacy organizations have formed with the mission of promoting equal rights for those with disabilities. These organizations work hard to educate the public about the challenges that people with fibromyalgia face. One of the primary goals of disability rights advocates is to ensure that people with fibromyalgia are not discriminated against in the workplace. Employers are required by law to provide reasonable accommodations for employees with disabilities. These accommodations can include flexible work schedules, ergonomic workstations, and additional breaks throughout the day to manage symptoms. It's crucial for those with fibromyalgia to be aware of their rights and advocate for themselves. Doing so can be overwhelming, but there are many resources available to help people with fibromyalgia navigate the complicated world of disability rights. Many disability rights organizations offer free legal services to help individuals with fibromyalgia understand the complex laws surrounding disability rights. In addition to educating oneself about disability rights, it's essential to spread awareness about fibromyalgia and the challenges faced by those who live with it. Sharing personal stories, writing letters to politicians, or participating in rallies for disability rights are all effective ways to raise awareness about fibromyalgia. It's important to remember that creating change takes time, and it's important to remain persistent in advocating for disability rights. Fibromyalgia is a debilitating condition that requires the support and understanding of society. Fighting for disability rights is essential for creating a society where people with fibromyalgia can participate fully. With perseverance, awareness, and education, we can work towards a future where disability rights are acknowledged and respected.

BUILDING A FIBROMYALGIA COMMUNITY

Living with fibromyalgia can be a lonely experience. Often, those who don't have first-hand experience with the condition struggle to understand it, leaving those with fibromyalgia feeling isolated and misunderstood. One of the best ways to combat this isolation is by building a community of people who truly understand what it's like to live with the invisible disability that is fibromyalgia.

Connecting with Others Online

The internet has made it easier than ever to connect with others who share your experiences. There are countless online communities dedicated to people living with chronic pain conditions like fibromyalgia, where you can find support, advice, and camaraderie. Social media platforms like Facebook and Twitter can also be great places to connect with others; you might try searching for groups or hashtags related to fibromyalgia and connecting with others that way.

Attending Fibromyalgia Events

Another great way to build community is by attending events that are specifically geared toward people with fibromyalgia. These might include support groups, educational workshops, or fundraisers for fibromyalgia research. Attending these events can help you connect with others who understand what you're going through, learn new coping strategies, and feel more empowered in your daily life.

Starting Your Own Community

If there aren't any existing fibromyalgia communities in your area, or if you're not finding what you need from the ones that exist, consider starting your own. This could be as simple as creating a Facebook group for people with fibromyalgia in your city or town, or as complex as organizing a full-fledged fibromyalgia awareness event. By taking the lead, you can create a supportive community that meets your needs and helps others in the same boat.

Building a Fibromyalgia Support Network

Whether you connect with others online, attend events, or start your own community, building a support network is an essential part of living well with fibromyalgia. These people will be there to offer you advice, encouragement, and understanding when you need it most. By building a strong community, you'll be better equipped to cope with the challenges of living with fibromyalgia and live a more fulfilling life overall.